Be Healed From High Blood Pressure
Stellah Mupanduki

Genre: Health, Self-Help, Body, Soul and Spirit, Christian Living, Books of Ministry.

Target Audience: All people: Male and female. Terminally ill people. Depressed people. Mentally ill people. Counselling groups. Synonymous groups. Outreach groups. Schools and Universities. Churches. Hospitals.

About the Book

Be Healed From High Blood Pressure is an anointed, powerful book for sacred healing, cleansing and protection from terminal illness, rare and all "incurable" diseases *of The heart and blood. It touches high blood pressure in a person's body and removes the controlling and chronic pressure. It removes all blood strongholds concerning the heart, brain, veins and arteries and bring peace to the body, mind and heart. It liberates the mind and body from living in the troubling state of dealing with chronic High Blood Pressure. This book is salvation to all people in different stages of life. It's a treasure that brings salvation to the mind, body and heart. If you are struggling with High and low blood pressure, do not worry anymore, this is your book of salvation from such diseases. Read and be well in the blood, veins, arteries and the heart and mind.*

Chapters

<u>Dedicated.</u>

To the whole world for the healing and protection of hearts
For the love of those who are suffering from heart diseases
To all those who seek true healing from God Almighty
To all those seeking personal healing and salvation
For the healing of the world that God created
To those who love to be have blessed hearts
For the peace of those hearts troubled
To the church and all families of God
For salvation of terminally ill people
For internal healing of the body
For the blessing of whole body
For sound Internal Organs.
To my children
Favour of God
Sound Family.
Romans 8:29-30
"For those God foreknew he also predestined to be conformed to the
likeness of his Son, that he might be the firstborn among many brothers.
And those he predestined, he also called; those he called, he also justified;
and those he justified, he also glorified."

Acknowledgement

Through Jesus Christ, Son of the Living God...These extraordinary books were written in the Truthful Leading, Healing, Guiding, Comforting, Pouring and Teaching of the Holy Spirit for the healing benefit of his people. No person or medical professional being, made any contribution to the writing of these books except the Holy Spirit himself using the author. He is the teacher and the healer and author of all mankind and creation. These books bring powerful intercession for healing before God on your behalf and allow you to communicate with the highest power in your life in a very free, calm, reassuring and fearless way. God is our best friend and Father full of love. As you read, you should smell the rich scent of the blood of Jesus Christ and as you close your eyes, you should see the cross where our Saviour died as a sign of your salvation.

Psalm 147:1 "Praise the LORD. How good it is to sing praises to our God, how pleasant and fitting to praise him."

For the Healing of Terminal illness, rare and incurable diseases books;

All in all, these powerful holy books are innovatively invented by God Almighty himself for the Healing of Terminal illness, rare and incurable diseases...they bring cleansing and protection to any person in this world. They take away brokenness, disgrace and hopelessness...they build up and they reconstruct...they mould everything...there is amazing Health Care and longevity...there are miracles and wonders...there is goodness and strength. Hallelujah! These books bring salvation through unique healing and peace to the people and all nations and all creation...They boost up every economy of every nation in this whole world. There is the solid truth about everything, there is divine love and compassion of God Almighty for his creation and people...Families are blessed with righteousness, blissful love, established stability, grace and peace from God Almighty in the name of Jesus Christ...There is blissful beauty, marvellous

growth, joy and happiness... In creating these books, God Almighty, the Holy Spirit uses the life of a woman who is his vessel of his presence, glory and honour in order to bring salvation and personal liberty and strength to all mankind and their surrounding...This whole world should praise and honour the Holy Spirit of the Sovereign God in all humbleness for his love and mercy...Hallelujah! "Thank you Father God...Thank you my Lord Jesus Christ...Thank you Holy Spirit...triune God...three in One...One in Three. I honour you...Maker of heaven and earth and everything in it...I love you from
Everlasting to Everlasting...Amen"

The Lord God Almighty said this to me; "Put these words of healing on paper as books...write them down so that my people will be healed and find peace in their lives and live longer..." And so this extra special gift of healing that is normally experienced on crusades is anointed and put on paper, written for the benefit of mankind and spread through the long and lasting, widespread book publishing industry. Man is mortal and I am a person who will come to cease existence from this world but the Word of God will remain for generations and generations and generations for the healing and salvation of mankind. Yeah...My time on earth as a vessel of God's glory and honour will come to an end when I am very, very, very old and grey and strong and powerful in the Lord...and I will go in his powerful glory. But the world will remain with all these unique books written by the Holy Spirit and operating in the healing, cleansing, protecting and saving presence of God himself.

- *"Nothing in these books should be added or subtracted..."* Says
the Lord God Almighty, who created heaven and earth.

NB: These Anointed and Sacred Healing For Terminal Illness, Rare and all Incurable diseases books will bring true, inclusive, holy, uniquely unique, pure, peaceful, stable, happy, exciting, interesting, gripping, comforting, stabilising and established, complete and permanent healing into your whole life and your family, your country, your continent and the whole world.

• Because of the Feeling of the Wounds of Christ, the Voice and the Sacred Heart of Christ in me; I am Uniquely Unique. Hallelujah.

Guidance

About Stellah Mupanduki

Healing For Terminal Illness Ministry:

Stellah Mupanduki of Jesus Christ...is a Charismatic Pentecostal Christian/*Interdenominational*... an Author, and has a miracle working Ministry for Spiritual healing for Terminal illness founded through the anointing power of the Holy Spirit. The essential principle she gives emphasis to and finds viable through her work is that there is hope for terminal illness and it is healed through Jesus Christ our Saviour. There is Hope for the hopeless. The Ministry is founded through a direct calling from God himself and operates in that realm of the Holy Spirit. She holds a Bachelors of Arts degree from the University of Zimbabwe(UZ) and a BCom (Specialising in Risk Management) from the University of South Africa (UNISA) and a Computer Business Application Specialist (Microsoft Office Certification) diploma. She has a liberating specific healing ministry that takes away desolation and death from those who can no longer be helped in the medical field. God is the answer when we are completely devoid of any ideas to help the hopeless. The Ministry takes away the grave, death sentences, fear, helplessness, disappointments and humiliation of untimely death by removing and eradicating diseases called terminal illness, rare and incurable diseases. Such diseases are now termed as historical because they are being removed and completely eradicated in the name of Jesus Christ.... For generations and generations until the ends of time, they are no more. Consider it done and finished. You do not have to worry anymore for *the Lord says this in the book of Isaiah 44: 24,26 "I am the Lord, your saviour; I am the one who created you. I am the LORD, the Creator of all things. I alone stretched out the heavens; when I made the earth, no one helped me......But when my servant makes a prediction, when I sent a messenger to reveal my plans, I make those plans and predictions come true."* GNB...

The Holy Spirit/Feeling of the wounds of Christ/Sacred heart is the greatest and unique person who has enabled the founder to operate and to write nervous system touching and healing, cleansing and protecting books that bring healing help to the hopeless and helpless depending upon his work and guidance that reaches out to the world. There is that holy divine purity in her work. And there is compassion and love for human life in these books. The love of music has helped her connect with the higher power of God that touches people and bring change in their lives. To be generous and kind at heart is a gift from God. Triune God as in God the Father, Son and the Holy Spirit. Three in One and One in three...Being used by God has made her realise how farreaching God`s love is through Jesus Christ our Saviour. For a person who is terminally ill, these books should be read on their own and should not be mixed with any other works of another person, great or unknown (small). Healing For Terminal Illness: Golgotha Hallelujah! Thank you Jesus Christ! Thank you Holy Spirit my Father, Jehovah Raphe, Almighty God, Holy One, Sovereign I AM...Hallelujah!

Other than life troubles in various areas of a person`s life, the Stellah Mupanduki books and personal presence give to the world a radical powerful healing, cleansing and protection from terminal illnesses, rare diseases and all controlling, incurable diseases. For Instance; *Cancers like; brain cancer, skin cancer, renal cancer, lung cancer, leukemia(Blood cancer), bladder cancer, uterine cancer, breast cancer, ovarian cancer, cervical cancer, prostate cancer, Oesophageal cancer, colorectal cancer, bile duct cancer, liver cancer, cancer of the pancreas, spleen cancer, bone cancer, bone marrow cancer, jaw cancer, cancer of the mouth, colon cancer, stomach cancer, cancer of the lymph nodes, throat cancer, cancer of the internal organs etc. ... for body, soul and mind healing, brain tumours, body tumours, Lung diseases, Chronic body pain...Alzheimer's, Multiple Sclerosis, Coma, Leukemia, Heart diseases, Heart attacks and Stroke, High and low blood pressure, Arthritis, Epilepsy, Parkinson, HIV/AIDS, Lupus, brain* diseases, Nervous system, internal organs, Progeria (Rare diseases), Asthma, Cystic fibrosis, Bones and marrow. The backbone, the Spine, obese, elephantiasis, Cholesterol, thrombosis, Diabetes, chronic stomach diseases, chronic incontinence, ulcers, anorexia, chronic depression, brain disorder-mental, neurological diseases...Cerebral Palsy, Sickle Cell Disease, leprosy...migraine, SIDS, skin diseases, osteoporosis, thyroid, Cysts, fibroids, veins and arteries, blood and genetic disorders, Dyslexia, ADD, Autism, down syndrome, sepsis, viruses, curses, allergies, eye diseases, mouth and ears: Speech problems, panic attacks, Cataracts, deaf and dumb, rare and incurable diseases, Barrenness: Womb healing; in matters of illness of the womb. Conceiving and protection from miscarriages........Substance abuse: Drug addiction...The Holy Spirit touches your body with his healing flow and heals all diseases in his supernatural way and ability.... My duty is to take everything the Holy Spirit of a Sovereign God is giving and I put it in writing for you to be healed and to fellowship with him...Hallelujah! Healing! Salvation!

NB: These Godly Invented Nerve Touching Healing Lullabies titles above took Me & the Holy Spirit, 8years of writing and editing. I was taught everything by the Holy Spirit of the Sovereign God himself. When he gave me the direction and command to publish these Healing lullabies books, he also gave me a dream of many stars in the dark sky; meaning, all people of all nations will be touched and healed in his name and power through these holy healing books....Just as the 10 Commandments were given to Moses by God Almighty; these healing lullabies are given directly from God Almighty to a woman, for the healing of nations and all people in the name of Jesus Christ...the Cross...You have to look at the cross and be healed in this era that we are living in this land of the living....God does not change and will never change nor matter what is done or what happens...The Spirit of God will always reveal himself in what he says and does.

Isaiah 40:3-5, "A voice of one calling; "In the desert prepare the way for the LORD; make straight in the wilderness a highway for our God. Every valley shall be raised up, every mountain and hill made low; the rough road shall become level, the rugged places a plain. And the glory of the LORD will *be revealed and all mankind will see it. For the mouth of the LORD has spoken.""" NIV Bible.*

Advice on how to Read the Lullabies Healing books invented by God Almighty for all his children on earth: And to all my readers, the presence of the Spirit of the Sovereign God is marked and felt by feelings felt during the process of reading. Hence you have to read them in your own private time when you are alone. Go into your reading room, your place of comfort and read as you lie down on your sofa, or just go into your bedroom, your solace, close your doors, lie down on your bed and just read and be touched in a deep and healing way by the Holy Spirit of a Sovereign God Almighty. Be in an undisturbed environment and enjoy the presence of God Almighty as you read and fellowship with him. Its all about you and the Holy Spirit.

And the *Healing Notes To the Readers of My Work is: The uniquely unique powerful presence of God you feel as you read my work is also the presence of the Holy Spirit you will feel when I am public speaking, teaching and ministering in your presence. And God makes me feel you as he heals you by touching my body with the healing touch you are receiving from him...There is nothing that God does not reveal to me his vessel of his presence, glory and honour...If he is healing breast cancer, he reveals to me...if he is touching strokes, he touches even one side of my body to show that someone with a right side stroke or left side stroke is being healed...he touches from the top of the head to the sole of the foot of that affected side...When he touches the brain, he reveals...When he goes to the heart, he shows this to me as well. He reveals his stabilising stability....When he touches the nerves and nervous system, he greatly touches me as well...he shows me...When he touches the lungs, he reveals...when he goes to the womb and all reproductive organs, he reveals...he reveals prostate cancer being healed by touching my abdomen as well...When he touches the spine, he reveals to me as well...He tells me who he is healing and what he is healing....And when he touches you from the top of your head with a strong grip and all the way to the soles of your feet, he also mercifully touches me with that healing flow you are receiving that feels like goose bumps on your skin...He touches your inner most being as well as my own inner-most being for me to be able to write and say this to you...Hence the recipient and the vessel of God have the same touch from the Almighty One for his glorification...We are all One in Christ, you and me...Hence I am able to praise him for you and me as well.*

Therefore, read these books without mixing them with any other person`s works except the Holy Bible itself, in its purity, that was breathed by the Spirit of God Almighty to the vessels who wrote it in days of old....No one in today's age should ever add or subtract anything in the Holy Bible by writing in it or commenting in it because commenting between lines or paragraphs in the bible will cause spiritual warfare to the reader no matter how powerful and well-known an author is...Respect the Holy Bible. Read the bible in its original form without any intrusion from people who write in it...This is not being selfish but helping you readers to receive pure and holy maximum healing from the Holy Spirit as he commands and speaks to your hearts in his purity, and for you to be able to give him the glory he deserves in order for him to pour himself out to the nations and people for more blessings...Benefit from the wounds of Christ and receive pure healing. This will work for you because there is true, complete and permanent healing from God Almighty, Maker of heaven and earth...Put 100% trust in God alone and you will be set free in permanent completeness... The Holy Spirit, the Spirit of the Sovereign God has poured out for you in order to be set free from all strongholds and I have put in writing everything he gave to you in these books.....Overcome the spirit of terminal illness, rare and incurable diseases...Purity! Safety! Healing! Protection! Hallelujah!

And the word of encouragement and truth I give about the Stellah Mupanduki books is that they should also be read to those who cannot read for themselves *because of illness*, or because of the fact that they are *babies* and those who are in a *Coma*...And to my able readers...As you read and absorb the prophetic healing words in these nervous system touching healing handiwork...you will experience the powerful supernatural healing presence of the Holy Spirit touching and healing your body inside and out. You will feel him on your skin and inside you...The healing Word in these books is about the *reader* and the Holy Spirit, it is about *you* and The Holy Spirit.

Holy...Holy: As you read these books, when you feel compelled to breathe his breath in ...do so...inhale his healing breath...make long and strong inhaling pulls...you will feel touched from the top of your head all the way to the soles of your feet...you will be touched on areas of your body that are troubling you...breathe in strongly and long and be healed. You will feel him touching you from the inside as you make these strong inhaling pulls...*Praise the Lord:* When you come on instances where the blood of Christ is mentioned and you start to choke, and cough or feel it in your throat, do not stop reading...keep going because anything bad in your body will be removed...keep reading do not be scared because you will be doing the right thing for your salvation...You are freed!

Hallelujah: When you feel your whole body filled with a soothing and cool wind...do not panic for God will be healing you in completeness....so let it be...*Holy:* When you feel compelled to be still and know he is God...go ahead and honour him through this anointing time of healing taking place in your body, put your book down and be quiet and still in body, just let go of yourself and allow the Holy Spirit of God to take control of your body, soul and spirit... *Glory:* When you feel compelled to keep reading...do so, keep absorbing because the Spirit of the Sovereign Lord is upon you helping you in this powerful healing journey. *Hosanna:* When you feel overwhelmed with his love and healing in your life and are compelled to praise Him and sing with Him and glorify His Name ...do so and be holy in his holiness...take the song that is put into your heart by the Holy Spirit himself and sing it in the way you love...*Praise the Lord!*

Thank you Lord: When you feel compelled to say out everything in your heart to him, do so, pour out all your feelings, your needs, your fears, your worries, your anger, your hurting, your loneliness in this time of affliction, say out whatever it is that you are going through when you feel compelled to do so...remove the death feeling from your soul ...*glory...glory...glory*...give everything to the Holy Spirit until you feel emptied of all burdens and your body, soul and mind feel light and relieved from burdens...just pour out your crying heart to the Lord God Almighty and he will answer you and heal you and comfort you in truth and in spirit....God Almighty will take away all rough patches in your life...He will remove all trials and all tribulations for you...the Lord who is your God will level your mountain...he will take all those burdens from you and you will never feel them or experience them in your life, and in your body, soul and mind again...Your life will be fine...the Lord Almighty will protect you from the negative throws of life...the Lord Almighty, the Sovereign I AM will remove all weakness from your life and you will truthfully overcome in great peace...there is healing for you...*Glory be to God Almighty.*

Hosanna: When there is a forceful continuous yawning, do not fight against the yawning...allow the yawning to go on until the Holy Spirit stops and you will feel very liberated and light in body...this is your key to your salvation...there is release of all evil and tension...the heavy burdens will be removed...you will feel the yawning strength and beauty in the healing that you will be experiencing...If you are reading to a child/baby; when they start this yawning process, shout Hosanna to God Almighty for true and permanent healing will be taking place, your child/baby will live ... *Cherubim... Cherubim... Hallelujah!*

Thank you Lord. When you feel warm in particular parts of your body, be happy...be relieved because God Almighty in the name of Jesus Christ is healing that part of your body...Finally when you feel his warmth wrapping around you and you need to sleep...put your book aside and sleep and feel nurtured as the healing flow of God Almighty spreads in your body in quietness...*Holy...holy...holy*

God Almighty: When you feel all weak in your body and you cannot do anything, and it feels like you are bound from doing anything for yourself...do not worry at all, it is all fine because God Almighty, will be breaking the illness and all evil for you......stay put, allow that weak and broken feeling in your body to prevail until you feel strong again. The Lord will give you that strength...you will be fine...you will regain strength!

Glory be to God Almighty...Salvation... Hallelujah: As you sleep, in the name of Jesus Christ, you will hear the helping voice of the Holy Spirit interceding on your behalf in your dreams...you will hear him praying for you and with you in his name...you will find yourself praying as you sleep dreaming dreams of your life and you wake up to realise that you were really praying facing a particular situation in your life e.g., dreams of someone in all black chasing you with a weapon, or some form of war where your life is at risk, or someone advancing at you in order to attack, or just being sick and helpless and in all this you overcome because you become very strong and vehement in prayer facing the warring situation...The Holy Spirit is living and active, emphatic and triumphant for you....You win...You will definitely love the Holy Spirit, the helper of your life, the Sovereign I AM...*Holy...holy...holy*! You will have wonderful healing and overcoming dreams of light, growth, the cross, water, the sun and moon and many more salvation dreams as given by the Holy Spirit himself to you...You will be renewed and refreshed when you wake up. You will regain strength and be filled with smiles because of the protecting and assuring divine helping presence of our merciful and forgiving God Almighty...*Glory!*

So as you finish reading these holy and sacred healing books, you will rise up because you will be set free. Jesus Christ came for you to be healed and be set free from all strongholds of life. Terminal illness, rare and incurable diseases can no longer scare you or make you live a fearful and uncertain life because there is healing in the name of Jesus Christ.

Healing!...Cleansing!...Salvation!...Protection!...Joy!...Hallelu jah!

Through his Name and blood, no life is left unchanged. God is merciful and loving to all. He is the Power in your life. And His healing flow in your body and his truthful presence will set you free as you read these sacred and holy books. Do not be afraid...read and find inner peace...Do not succumb to discouragement, troubles and death... There is healing coming from God Almighty to you... There is no one like our God...*Beautiful Hallelujah! Hosanna! Amen.*

Powered by the Finger of God...Holy Spirit...Living and Active.(Guidance on Reading is put in every new manuscript produced)

Isaiah 44: 23 "Shout for joy, you heavens. Shout, deep places of the earth! Shout for joy, mountains and every tree of the forest! The LORD has shown his greatness by saving his people Israel"
GNB.

<u>Chapter 1</u>

Heart At Peace

Isaiah 52:8-10

"Listen! Your watchmen lift up their voices; together they shout for joy. When the LORD returns to Zion, they will see it with their own eyes. Burst into songs of joy together, you ruins of Jerusalem, for the LORD has comforted his people, he has redeemed Jerusalem. The LORD will lay bare his holy arm in the sight of all the nations, and all the ends of the earth will see the salvation of our God."

> * I speak healing and restoration in your body in the powerful name of the Lord Jesus Christ. Be healed from High Blood Pressure...be healed in your heart...be well in your veins and arteries...be well in the blood that flow in your veins...be at peace in your blood...be healed in the wonderful name of the Lord Jesus Christ...In the powerful power of the Holy Spirit; I speak life to your veins and arteries...I speak goodness to your heart...I speak healing to your veins and arteries...I speak protecting to your body and brain...I speak salvation from High Blood
> Pressure...I speak life to you in that glorious name above every name...Be healed from hypertension in the name of the Lord Jesus Christ. Be healed from hypertension...be healed in that wonderful name of Jesus...I command the illness of high and low blood pressure to get out of your veins and arteries...I command the spirit of hypertension to get out of your

heart, blood vessels and life...I command it to go in the powerful name of the Lord Jesus Christ. Be at peace...Be in good shape...be healthy in your body, soul and spirit...Be healed in your heart, veins and muscles...be healed from aneurysm...may the Lord completely protect your arteries from being enlarged...may the good Lord protect your arteries from busting...be protected from haemorrhoids...be strong and secure in your veins and arteries...be healed in your blood...be at peace in your blood, veins and arteries...be healed in that wonderful name of the Lord Jesus Christ...Take comfort...Be well again...do not be afraid...may the Lord heal you from the spirit of phobia in the powerful and saving name of the Lord Jesus Christ. Be healed from shock and panic attacks...be healed and be at peace...I speak salvation to you in that wonderful name of the Lord Jesus Christ who redeemed your life.

John 8:32
"Then you will know the truth, and the truth will set you free."

* Holy Father, I come before you in the depth of my heart...help me to know and see the truth that will set me free...show your glory in my life...Reveal the things that are bringing confusion to my life and heal me...Make a straight path for me...level my path...remove all rough patches from my body and life...raise the valleys for me Lord...lift me up to your goodness...remove every mountain and hill from the path of my life...make any crooked road of my life straight for me...level the path that I am walking...heal me Lord...heal my heart, body and mind...heal my life for me and make everything well for me...show me my

road of truth and let me travel that journey of my life in your truthful presence, mercy and love. Hold my hand and walk with me Lord...be with me all the time...protect me from the spirit of demise...Heal me Lord...Remove obstacles from the path of my life...Remove disease of old age from my body...remove high blood pressure from my veins and arteries...remove low blood pressure from my veins and arteries...remove heart troubles from my physical heart...remove all sorrows that cause destruction to my heart...purify my blood from all impurities...save me from strokes and heart failures...protect my brain and heart...protect my body...keep me healthy in every part of my body...keep me safe in your protecting presence...bring complete and permanent healing to my body and soul...protect me from being afflicted from terminal illness and all diseases...remove all brokenness from my heart and body and blood...make me healthy and secure in my body and mind...immerse me in the precious blood of my Lord Jesus Christ...Make me well again, Lord...make my body curable...remove all chronic pain of the heart and body...remove struggles of my heart...give me your peace and quietness...make me well again...remove all desperation and take me away from succumbing into desperate measures of seeking healing...I belong to you Lord...heal me Lord...Make me physically fit all the days of my life...cleanse and protect me with your healing flow in my body, heart and blood...make me strong...do good things for me...Touch my heart and heal me from pain and suffering...remove all constriction of the heart...make my heart flexible and peaceful...Bless my heart with endurance and strength...Breathe stability into my body, mind and heart...protect me from the spirit of demise...I am your child...show your truthful love to me your wonderful child who loves you...help me to live against all odds and worship you in all humbleness and goodness. Touch my heart with your presence dear Father and let your light shine through my body and life in the name of the Lord Jesus Christ my Redeemer. Make those who are around me be honest and faithful...give me peace in my heart...protect my soul and heart from being broken...Surround me with your goodness and mercy...remove all physical and emotional abuse from touching my heart and life...Touch those around me with all your goodness and love...Make them righteous in all their ways and bless the words that come from their mouths...Bring good health to their minds and ways...heal their bodies and hearts with your goodness...You are our God of peace and love...nothing is hidden from you Lord

Almighty...all that we do is laid bare before you...Lead us to all your truth through your Holy Spirit that dwell in us...help us to do the right things in our lives...Help us to stay in the truth and to be true before you and to ourselves...You are the Lord God Almighty who knows the thoughts and attitudes of human hearts and you are the one who judges the thoughts and attitudes of our human hearts' through our desires...help us to be true... help us to come clean and healed in the hearts...set us free from sin with your truth that gives eternal life in the name of the Lord Jesus Christ...Heal us Lord...heal us your children...heal your flock...be with us always...bless our lives with your powerful and protecting presence...give us your grace and peace through your Holy Spirit...protect us Holy One,

Sovereign I AM...Immerse us in the sacred and sanctifying blood of your precious Son Jesus Christ, the Lamb of God who took away the sins of the world.

Psalm 69:20

"Scorn has broken my heart and has left me helpless; I looked for sympathy, but there was none, for comforters but I found none."

* Peace to your mind and heart! The Lord is with you always. He is protecting you. You are above and not beneath. The Lord is removing all those things that brought ridicule in your life. The Lord is removing those instruments of ridicule from tormenting you. The Lord is crushing those who ridicule you. The Lord God Almighty is your comfort. He is mending and healing your heart in the name of the Lord Jesus Christ. He is giving you his strength, love and respect through a good placing and restoration. You are the head and not the tail. You will never fail. You are a success. The good Lord who created you is making things right for you. The Lord has compassion for you and he knows where he is taking you. He is taking you to a good place for his name's sake and you will be fine. You are secure. You are safe and sound. Those who poured derision upon your life and circumstances are removed from your path and can only watch you from afar. They can only hear about your success and fail to come near. The good Lord is making you strong in the highest name of the Lord Jesus Christ. He is the only power that can give you the best for your life in truthfulness and honesty. In your weakness he makes you strong. He gives purpose to your life. Do not be worried any more.

Everything happens for a reason and that reason is good for your life and it holds together for you through Jesus Christ. You will breakthrough. You are in this situation for the sake of the glory of the Lord, for the sake of his goodness in this world. You are already stepping forward in the name of the Lord Jesus Christ. Be at peace he will raise you up.

Habakkuk1: 12
"O LORD, are you not from everlasting? My God, my Holy One, we will not die."
You will not die...

* In the name of Jesus Christ, in the powerful blood of Christ, you will not die, you live to glorify the name of the Lord Almighty who heals you...it is not yet time for you to depart from this land of the living...the Lord Almighty says this to you my dear friend; *"Be healed in your body...be healed in your inmost being. Be healed from illness. Be set free from the stronghold of terminal illness. Be healed in your heart. Be healed and be protected with an everlasting protection. Be at peace in your body, soul and mind...be protected from struggling in your heart...be at rest in the heart...be healed from chronic pain in the heart...be healed my dear child...be healed with peace in your heart...be firm and steadfast in the heart...be holy in your heart...be healed from strokes...be healed from heart attacks...be saved in your heart and mind...be holy in my holiness...be healed in your life...be protected in my glory and honour...be healed with an everlasting healing...be healed from pain...be healed from suffering...be healed from all struggles in the heart...fear not for I am with you and in you...be healed in my presence...I love you my child...you belong to me...be healed in my power and strength...Overcome all trials and tribulations...be at peace...be able to endure...be strong in the heart for I am with you*

and in you...be triumphant in everything...conquer all evil in my name and power for I am with you and in you...Be strong in your heart, soul and body...be strong in your mind for I am with you and in you...You breakthrough my beloved one...you overcome in my healing presence...I am the Lord the Almighty One who helps you and sustains your life...you are mine and I will not forsake you...Be at peace and in peace all the days of your life...Be healed in your heart...be healed with a permanent and everlasting healing flow...be healed my child...be healed because I love you...be healed because I am your God and you are my child...be healed in my peace...Do not be troubled anymore...do not fail in the heart...do not struggle in your heart my dear child...I, the Lord, the Almighty One am with you , helping you all the days of your life for I live with you and in you...you are mine...be healed in your heart... be healed my dear child...You live...you overcome...you break through in my name and powerful presence...I will never forsake you...be healed in your heart...You have a hope and a future. Everything is fine with you...It is well with your heart and soul." ...Says the Sovereign I AM.

Thank you Lord, thank you Holy One... Thank you Holy Spirit, my Everlasting Father... Glory be to your name forever and ever.

* Hallelujah: Dear Reader, you will live long because the Lord who is your God has said so, the Almighty One has healed your life, the Sovereign I AM has blessed you with a wonderful healing in the name of the Lord Jesus Christ...God wants you to live very long...God wants you to live a healthy and normal life...God is removing chronic illnesses from your life...God Almighty is eradicating high blood pressure...God almighty is removing the spirit of high and low blood pressure from your body and life...be healed in his power...Glory be to God Almighty, you

live your life in peace...You will not die at all. Your heart will not die. Your mind will not die...Your body will not die...Your heart is made wholesome and durable...be healed in the powerful name of the Lord Jesus Christ...The Lord is your shepherd and you shall not be in want...he leads you to quiet waters and refreshes your soul. He heals and revives your heart...Be healed from high blood pressure...be healed from a chronic illness...be set free from a fatal stronghold...be healed from living with high blood pressure...be set free in the healing power of God Almighty who created heavens and earth, seas and oceans, rolling rivers and lakes and everything in them...be healed in his powerful power...be healed from high blood pressure...be healed from uncertainty...be well in your heart, brain, veins and arteries...be protected from bursting in the arteries and veins...be protected from hemorrhoids...be healed from high blood pressure...be well in your veins and arteries...be well in your heart...Live long...have power in the heart...be healed in the wonderful name of the Lord Jesus Christ, the Lamb of God who took away the sins of the world...May the Lord God Almighty hold your heart in peaceful healing...May he protect your heart from being robbed of life...be healed in his saving name...be healed from the top of your heart, be healed all the way to the bottom of your heart...be healed from the North to the South of your heart...be healed from the East to the West of your heart...be immersed in the healing power of the living and active God Almighty, who is mighty to save and to protect...Let your heart rest in his supernatural healing presence...let your heart be completely immersed in the saving and protecting blood of the Lord Jesus Christ, the Lamb of God who took away the sins of the world...Be healed and find peace in your heart and body...be healed in the arteries...be healed and be strong in your veins...May the good Lord cleanse you according to his promises of healing in your life. Yes, be healed in his righteous name... be able bodied my good friend...have a sound body, have a sound heart, have a sound mind...be healed in that precious name of the Lord Jesus Christ...Hallelujah! Thank you Holy Spirit.

Psalm 28:7

"The LORD is my strength and my shield; my heart trusts in him, and I am helped. My heart leaps for joy and I will give thanks to him in song."

* Be healed in the heart; be artistic...be aware of things...have good insight...understand...distinguish...be focused in the mighty name of the Lord Jesus Christ...Be healed from heart stroke in that saving name of the Lord Jesus Christ...Be healed from pain in the heart...be healed from weakness of the heart...be healed from all heart failure...Regain strength in his wonderful name...have ability to move on your own...be revived in the Lord...have ability in joints and muscle, fibre, tissues and all cells...rise up and walk in the healing name of the Lord Jesus Christ. Be healed from pain and tiredness in the name of the Lord Jesus Christ. Have the strength to speak...be able to sing... dance in the name of the Lord Jesus Christ...move again in the powerful name of the Lord Jesus Christ...May the Lord God Almighty bath you with his healing presence and comfort you in the powerful name of the Lord Jesus Christ.

Psalm 86:3-4

"Have mercy on me, O LORD, for I call to you all day long. Bring joy to your servant, for to you, O LORD, I lift up my soul."

> *"I love you my child, be healed from internal bleeding...be healed in veins and arteries...be healed...be healed from heart failure...Do not be sick in the heart...Succeed...Overcome for I am with you."* Says the Lord your God.

> *Dear Reader, submit to God and say, "I love you God. I love you Jesus Christ. I love you Holy Spirit. I am safe and secure in you and with you. I have strength and confidence in you and I am able to move in your power and help...You are my sure support and my shield...You are always with me Lord and I rise in your power and in your name. I am not afraid anymore."

Psalm 16:9, 10

"Therefore my heart is glad and my tongue rejoices; my body will also rest secure, because you will not abandon me to the grave, nor will you see your Holy One see decay."

> *May the good Lord heal and protect you from heart stroke...may he kindly protect you from brain damage...be healed from high blood pressure...be protected from high blood pressure...be protected from the top of your head and all the way to the soles of your feet...be protected from failure of the heart...be healed from high blood pressure...be healed and protected in the name of the Lord Jesus Christ. Be healed in the brain...be healed from all forms of illness of the brain, heart, veins and arteries...be healed from brain cancer...be healed from brain tumours...be protected in your brain...be healed from the spirit of rare diseases of

the brain...may there be peace in the heart, blood, veins and arteries and the brain and body...be healed from all chronic illness of the heart and brain...be healed from high blood pressure...be healed from chronic pain in your mind...be healed from chronic headaches...be healed in your nervous system...be healed in your nerves...be healed in all your motor skills...be stable in your body...may God our Father protect you from losing balance and falling...be healed from high blood pressure...be healed in your heart...be healed in your veins...be healed in your arteries...be healthy in your blood flow... be cured from high blood pressure...be cured from illness of the heart, blood, veins and arteries...be healed in your body...have stability of body, soul and mind...be healed your innermost being...be healthy in your heart...be healthy in your body...be healed in every part of your brain...be protected in the brain...may the healing flow of God protect you brain, heart and body with his goodness...may the Lord protect the mind from being destroyed...be completely healed in all your brain lobes...be healed with a sound and healthy frontal lobe...be at peace in your temporal lobe...be intact in the parietal lobe...be completely healed in the occipital lobe...be safe and sound in all your brain lobes...be protected in every brain lobe...be normal in the brain...function well in your brain...be healed from illness in the brain...be stable and peaceful in your brain...be well in your brain...be healed in your heart and brain...be protected from illness of the brain...be immersed in the saving and protecting blood of the Lord Jesus Christ...Be protected from the spirit of seizures, coma, and loss of brain parts...be protected from strokes...be healed from high blood pressure...be healed in the brain...be intact in your brain...May the good Lord keep all your brain lobes intact...may he breathe his healing breath in all your brain lobes...Be healed in the brain...be healed with goodness and strength in your brain...be healed with good ability in your brain...be rational in your brain...function well in every part of your brain...be healed from illness of the brain...be healed in that wonderful name of the Lord Jesus Christ...May God Almighty in all his care and love heal and protect you in the mind...be healed in the spinal code...be healed with strength in your spinal code and all spinal fluid...Be healthy in the mind and body...be healed from the spirit of illness...be healthy in every part of your body...Hallelujah; be healed your cerebellum...be healed in completeness in your cerebrum...be healed in all your brain stem...be protected in the mind...be saved from troubles of the mind...be healed my good friend...be protected from the effects of high blood pressure...be healed and have a healthy brain...be secure in the brain...be logical...be conscious...be alert...be stable in the brain...have good balance in your brain...be healed with good memory...be completely healed in your mind...have good balance...be healed with a good self-control of your emotions...be healthy in your brain...be set free from being eroded in the brain...be healed from all brain injury...be immersed in that wonderful blood of the Lord Jesus Christ...Be healed with good and powerful motor skills...be protected in the mind...be completely protected with the power of the Living God who is mighty to save you...be healed in his healing power...be healed with a permanent healing from God Almighty, Maker of heavens and earth...Be protected in all four winds...be protected from the North to the South and from the East to the West of your brain...be wholesomely protected in your brain...be powerfully healed and protected in your brain...Be sealed in the precious and saving blood of the Lord Jesus Christ...Be healed in your mind...be healed in every part of your brain...be healed in completeness...may there be a good flow of blood and oxygen in your brain...may the good Lord touch all your nerves and revive you...may God Almighty bring good co-ordination to your motor skills and heal you in completeness...may the Almighty One touch your sensory nerves and restore and revive them...be healed from injury in the brain...be set free from brain damage...be mended in your brain...be healed with wonderful and perfect motor skills...Be able to see...be able to speak...be able to reason...be able to have good taste...be able to feel...be able to hear...be physically sound...remember...have a wonderful memory...be strong in the mind...be healthy in every part of your mind...be healed in the name of the Lord Jesus Christ...Hallelujah; may the good Lord protect your sensory nerves in that powerful name of the Lord Jesus Christ...be healed in your brain...be healed in your body...be healed permanently...be healed in sweetness and power...be completely healed in that glorious name of our Lord Jesus Christ...Rise up...read and write...have a good grip...be normal again in the prevailing name of the Lord Jesus Christ.

*Dear Reader; honour God Almighty, Everlasting Father and say; "You are my Holy God who brings relief to my soul, mind and body. Lift me up and give me your goodness on this earth and breathe in your everlasting life when my life on this earth has come to an end according to your will. Heal my body in your mercy and love...Heal me Lord. Restore me. Revive me as your child through Jesus Christ your first born."

Psalm 105:2-4

"Sing to him, sing praise to him; tell of all his wonderful acts. Glory in his holy name; let the hearts of those who seek the LORD rejoice. Look to the LORD and his strength; seek his face always."

*I speak joy in your life in the name of the Lord Jesus Christ. I speak peace and long life to you in the power of the Holy Spirit. I speak protection in the heart...I speak the Lord`s favour for your heart and mind...I speak healing in your life...I speak healing to your internal organs...be healed in your heart...be healed in your veins and arteries...be healed in the blood that flow in your veins and arteries...be well in your blood form...be healthy in your blood type...be healed from illness of the blood...be healed from high blood pressure...be healed from low blood pressure...be well connected to the body organs in blood, veins and arteries...be healed in your pancreas...be healed from blood glucose...be healed from the spirit of diabetes...be healed in the name of the Lord Jesus Christ...Be well in your pancreas...be well in your mind...be well in your blood...be purified in your blood...be healthy in your veins and arteries...be healed from diabetes...be healed from the spirit of blood sugar...be healed in your body, heart and pancreas...be healed in every part of your heart...be healed in your body and mind...be completely healed in that wonderful name of the Lord

Jesus Christ...Be well in your pancreas...be cured from chronic illness of the pancreas...be cured from the spirit of diabetes...be protected from diabetes...be healed in that wonderful name of the Lord Jesus Christ...be set free from the stronghold of diabetes...be healed in your flesh and blood...be healthy in the blood that flow in your veins and arteries...have good blood circulation in your veins and arteries and heart...be healed in your heart...be healed in your internal organs...be restored to goodness in your pancreas...be well in your motor skills...be restored to goodness in your eyes...be healed from losing eyesight...be healed in your eyes...be protected in your motor skills...be protected in your sensory nerves...be healed in your body...be well coordinated in the body, heart, pancreas and the brain...be healed with goodness in your body, soul and spirit...be healed in your brain...be set free from slipping into a coma...be healthy in your heart, pancreas, blood, brain and sensory nerves...be healed through the powerful power of God Almighty...be healed in your body...be healed from diabetes...be healed from pain in the heart...be healed with a complete and permanent healing in your pancreas...be healed from all pancreas diseases...be healed in goodness...diabetes is bound from prevailing in your body...diabetes is eradicated from your body...it is hindered from prospering in your body...it is cut-off...it is completely removed from your body...it is wiped out from your body...the Lord Almighty eradicates the spirit of diabetes from this planet...it is no more...the spirit of infirmity is bound from prevailing...it is wiped away from your body...it is bound from prevailing in your body...it is sent to Hades where it belongs and it will never return again...you are set free from the spirit of diabetes...you are removed from the clutches of diabetes...every type and form of diabetes is removed from this planet...it is eradicated...it is removed from oppressing you and all people...it is removed from your body...you are healed in your pancreas...you are healed in your blood...you are healed in your heart...you are healed from high blood pressure...you are healed from diseases of the heart and blood and blood vessels...you are healed in all your internal organs...you are set free from all illness of the pancreas...you are healed from illness of the heart and blood vessels...you are healed in your body...you are healed and set free from the clutches of the spirit of infirmity...you are fully immersed in the saving and protecting blood of the Lord Jesus Christ, the Lamb of God who took away the sins of the world...You are healed from bloodline diseases...you removed from the clutches of genetic blood diseases...you are healed from the stronghold of high blood pressure...you are healed from low blood pressure...you are healed from chronic illness...you are healed and protected from terminal illness of the blood, veins and arteries...You are healed on your skin...you are set free from the spirit of wounds...yeah, be healed in completeness...be healed from the top of your head and all the way to the soles of your feet...be healed with good health all the days of your life...be well in your pancreas...be well in your blood...be well in flesh and blood...be well in your brain...be well in all your nerves...be well in your nervous system...be well in your motor skills...be wholesome in your sensory nerves...be healthy in your heart...be healed with a complete healing coming from God Almighty who created you...be healed from diabetes...be healed with stability in your body and blood...be well in all your internal organs...be healed in your heart...be healed in the blood that flow in your veins and arteries...be healed from pressure...be healed from constriction of the veins and arteries...be healed from tightness of the heart...be well in your heart...be healthy in every part of your heart...be at peace in your heart, blood, veins and arteries...be healed from head aches...breathe well...be healed from all pain...be efficient in the pancreas...be sufficient in your pancreas...have ability in your pancreas...be healed from the stronghold of a chronic illness...be healed from diabetes...it is removed from your life...be protected from the spirit of illness...be protected from the top of your head and all the way to the soles of your feet...be protected from the spirit of numbness of the soles of your feet...be healed from poor blood circulation...be protected from numbness of toes and feet...be healed from diabetes and all illness...it is fully conquered...it is removed from troubling your body...you live long...you are freed from living a controlled life...be healed in your body...be protected from the spirit of numbness in your fingertips... be healed from the spirit of sharp pricking's in your feet and body...be healed in your heart...be healed in your veins and arteries...be healed from illness of the blood, veins and arteries...be healed in every part of your heart...have good flow and circulation of blood in your veins and arteries all over your body, from the top of your head and all the way to the soles of your feet...be well in your heart valves...be well in your heart chambers...be well in in blood texture...be well in blood flowing in your veins and arteries...be healed from blood clotting...be healed from opaque…be healed from bad cholesterol…be healed in your veins and arteries…be healed from blocked veins and arteries…be healed in every part of your heart…be efficient in your heart…be healed from the spirit of infirmity…be healed…be healed…be healed with a wonderful healing flow of God Almighty touching you from the top of your head and flowing all the way to the soles of your feet with a wonderful healing flow…be healed in your heart with a complete healing flow coming from God Almighty Maker of heaven and earth, seas and oceans, rolling rivers and waterfalls and lakes and everything in them…be healed in the mercy of God Almighty who created you and who has the supernatural powerful power to heal you with a permanent healing in his everlasting ways...be well in your body...be set free from the stronghold of sharp needles and pricking in your body...be healed from all body pain…be healed in your brain...be healed from illness...be protected from coma...be living and active in the heart, blood, veins, arteries, brain and body...be alert in your brain...be logical...be protected in your heart and brain...be protected from the spirit of demise...be protected from high blood pressure…be protected from low blood pressure…be healed in your blood, veins and arteries…be healed in your heart and body…be well in all your internal organs…have good blood circulation in your body…be protected from strokes…be healed from heart attacks…be healthy in your heart, blood, veins and arteries…be healed from high and low blood pressure…be set free from the spirit of hypertension…be well in your body, heart and mind...be protected in your pancreas and brain...be healed in your lungs…be able to breathe well in your

lungs all the days of your life…be efficient in your heart,
veins, arteries, lungs and brain all the days of your
life…be protected in your flesh and blood...be healed
with strength in your body...be protected from the spirit
of fainting...be alert and energetic...be healed from
illness...be healed in your body... be healed from
diabetes...be healed from autoimmune diseases…be
well in your blood vessels…be healthy in your blood
circulation…be protected from collapsing veins and
arteries…be protected from blocked veins and
arteries…be protected from blocked heart valves…be
healed in your heart…be healed with a complete and
permanent healing of the blood and heart…be
protected from illness of the blood and blood
vessels…be healed in that wonderful name of the Lord
Jesus Christ…Be healed from the spirit of
haemorrhage…be healed from raptured veins and
arteries…be healed from aneurysm…be healed in your
veins and arteries…be healed from high blood
pressure…be healed in your heart and body…be healed
in your heart muscles…be healed from the spirit of
strokes and heart failure…be fully immersed in that
saving and protecting blood of the Lord Jesus Christ,
the Lamb of God who took away the sins of the
world…Yeah, be healed in the name of our Lord Jesus
Christ…Be healed from high blood glucose…be healed
in the blood…be well in the blood…be balanced in
your blood…be set free from pressures of the
blood…be healed in that inmost being….be healed
from diseases of the blood and blood vessels…be
healed from leukemia…be healed from diabetes…be
healed from autoimmune diseases…be healed from
viruses…be well in the blood…be stable in the heart,

blood and blood vessels…be set free from the spirit of infirmity…Be healed from diabetes…diabetes is no more…it is gone to Hades where it belongs…it is removed from your body once and for all…you are well in your pancreas and blood…you are well in your heart, veins, arteries, blood and pancreas…you are well in your body…you are cleansed in your blood…you are well in your mind…you are well in your flesh and blood…be healed from illness…be healed in your pancreas…be healed from pancreatitis…be healed from cancer of the pancreas…be healed with goodness in your pancreas…be healed from failure of the pancreas…be well again in your pancreas and body…be well in your brain…be well in in the blood that flow all over your body through your veins and arteries…be well in the heart that pumps the blood that flow in your body through your veins and arteries…be healthy in your body and heart…be healed through the healing power of God Almighty, Maker of heaven and earth, seas and oceans, rolling rivers and lakes and everything in them…be healed with his cleansing healing…be healed from the top of your head and all the way to the soles of your feet…be healed from illness…be healed with goodness…be healed…be healed…be healed…be well again… Be healed in that supreme name of the Lord Jesus Christ…Be at peace in your heart…be secure in your vital heart for the Lord is healing and protecting you all the days of your life…be healed from high blood pressure…be healed from low blood pressure…be healed from all blood infections…be healed from viral infections of the blood and heart…be healed in your body…be at peace in your heart and brain…be at peace in your body…be stable in the heart and body…be strong in your heart and body...be well in the heart, body and mind...be healed in that powerful name of the Lord Jesus Christ...Hallelujah!

Psalm 147: 3
"He heals the broken-hearted and binds up their wounds."

*Be whole again in the name of the Lord Jesus Christ. Be healed in your respiratory system. May the good Lord heal your heart...May he mend all brokenness in the heart. May he bring healing to the heart valves. May our Lord God Almighty, in his sacredness heal you from coronary artery diseases...Be healed from high blood pressure...be healed in your veins and arteries...be healed in the blood that flow in your veins...be healed with goodness in your heart and body and mind...be healed with peace...be healed with stability in your veins and arteries and the blood that flow in them... be purified in the blood that flow in your veins and arteries...be healthy in your heart, veins and arteries...be healthy in your blood...be healed from illness of the heart, blood, veins and arteries...be healed through the powerful power of God Almighty...Be healed in that wonderful name of the Lord Jesus Christ...May the good heal your blood from high cholesterol...may the Almighty One iron out bad cholesterol from your heart and blood and veins...be healed in your body...be healed in your flesh and blood...Be healed from the top of your head and all the way to the soles of your feet...be healed with a powerful healing flow of God Almighty, Maker of heaven and earth...be healed in that powerful name of the Lord Jesus Christ...Hallelujah...May the Lord Almighty in his supreme ways remove and defeat obesity and overweight from the body...be healed in your flesh and blood...Be healed in the healing name of the Lord Jesus Christ...May the good Lord remove all stress from your life...may he heal your body from diabetes...Be completely healed in that good name of our Lord Jesus Christ...Be healed from loss of hearing...be healed from loss of sight...be healed from loss of speech, be healed in your motor skills...be healed in all your nerves...be completely healed in your nervous system...be healed from the top of your head and all the way to the soles of your feet...be healed with goodness in your body...be healed through the healing flow of God Almighty who sees you...be healed in truth and in spirit...be healed from strokes...be healed from heart attacks...be living and active in the heart...be healthy in your body, heart and mind...be protected from the spirit of demise...be protected from heart failure...be well in your heart and mind...be well in your body and spirit...be immersed in that saving and protecting blood of the Lord Jesus Christ, the Lamb of God who took away the sins of the world...Be strong in your heart...be well established in your heart...be at peace in your heart...be stable in your heart all the days of your life...Hallelujah; be healed with a permanent healing from God Almighty...Be healed in the glorious name of the Lord Jesus Christ.

Psalm 30:8-10

"To you, O LORD, I called; to the Lord I cried for mercy: "What gain is there in my destruction, in my going down into the pit? Will the dust praise you? Will it proclaim your faithfulness? Hear, O LORD, and be merciful to me; O LORD, be my help.""

*Be healed and protected from the spirit of cardiac arrest...be healed in the powerful name of the Lord Jesus Christ. May the Lord restore and revive your heart...May the Lord almighty, Maker of heaven and earth cover and protect your heart with the saving and healing blood of the Lord Jesus Christ...May the grace and peace of our Lord Jesus Christ be with you...may he uphold you...may he carry you through...may he give joy to your heart...may he shield your brain and body from death and disintegration...be healed in his healing name...be healed in the name above every name...be healed from the spirit of high blood pressure...be at peace in your blood...be at peace in the blood vessels that carry your blood...be at peace in your heart....be healed in the name of the Lord Jesus Christ. May the Lord God Almighty restore you to perfection...may he make your form and frame upright...may he bless your body, mind and spirit with the ability to grow in his glorious and healing name...May he give good and strong form to your bone structure...may he make you straight and not bowed...may he give continuous strength to your bones...may he give you good support...may he make you normal again in the name above every name...that wonderful name of the Lord Jesus Christ.

Psalm 69:5
"You know my folly, O God; my guilty is not hidden from you."

*The Lord your God is a God of forgiveness...he restores you to righteousness...be healed in his glorious name...may the Lord touch your heart and heal you in his righteous ways...May the Lord God Almighty be

merciful to you in the name of the Lord Jesus Christ.
Be happy in your veins and arteries...be healed from
constriction of the veins and arteries...be well in your
blood...be healed from high blood pressure...be healed
from low blood pressure...be well in your blood, veins
and arteries...be well in your heart...be at peace in your
brain...be healed from chronic high blood pressure...be
healed from chronic low blood pressure...be normal in
your blood flow...be healed in power...be healed with
the healing flow of God Almighty flowing in your
blood...be healed from the spirit of high blood
pressure...be healed in the name of Jesus Christ...Be
healed in his power and majesty in the name of the Lord
Jesus Christ. Be strong...be confident...receive life...be
at peace before his throne of grace and receive freely
from him who atoned for your transgressions...be set
free from the stronghold of high blood pressure...be
protected from strokes and heart attacks...have a good
level of blood...be healed from high blood pressure...be
healed in your heart...Be healed in the name that is
above every name...be healed in the name of Jesus
Christ...Be healed in his righteous name...High blood
pressure is broken, it is wiped out from your heart,
veins and arteries...high blood pressure is cut off...high
blood pressure is no more...the Lord who is the Creator
of heavens and earth, seas and oceans, rolling rivers,
waterfalls and lakes and everything in them, is a healing
and merciful God...there is nothing impossible for
him...be healed in his power...be healed in your
heart...be healed in your blood flow...be healed in your
veins and arteries...be well in your body and heart...be
healed from chronic pain of the mind...be healed from
the incontrollable high blood pressure...be healed in

that wonderful and powerful power of God Almighty...be good in your body, soul and mind...be at peace all the days of your life...be set free from living with a chronic illness...be set free from the stronghold of high blood pressure...be healed in that powerful name of the Lord Jesus Christ...Hallelujah; thank you Jesus Christ my Saviour...thank you for the cross that has brought salvation to mankind and all creation...Hallelujah.

Proverbs 11:20
"The LORD detests men of perverse heart but he delights in those whose ways are blameless."

*Be healed in the desires of your heart...be healed with wisdom and peace in the longing of your heart...be holy in the heart...be healed from all heart murmurs...be healed from all heart conditions...do not complain in the heart...do not cry in the heart...be healed in your heart...be healed from all illness of the heart...be healed from chronic pain of the heart...be healed from all chronic illness of the heart...be strong and healthy in your heart...be healed from terminal illness of the heart...be set free from the clutches of rare diseases of the heart...be healed in your heart, body and mind...be healed with goodness and love...be healed with joy and happiness in your heart...be healthy in your heart...be at peace in your heart...be healed with love and honour in your heart...be blessed with a good heart in everything that you do...Be healed through the healing power of God Almighty who is Maker of heaven and earth...be healed in that wonderful name of the Lord Jesus Christ...Be strong in your body and heart...be strong in your life...be blessed with a good heart...be healed and be blessed with a remorseful heart...be beautiful in everything that you do and say...be open-minded and be open-hearted in all your dealings...be beautiful in the heart and mind...be immersed in the precious blood of the Lamb of God who took away the sins of the world...be protected from heart attacks...be protected from failing in the heart...be healed from all troubles of life...be surrounded with the protecting presence of God Almighty...be protected in your life and body...be freed from all strongholds in the heart...be healed in your heart...be completely healed in the name of the Lord Jesus Christ.

Proverbs 17: 22
A cheerful heart is good medicine, but a crushed spirit dries up the bones."

* Be blessed with salvation in the heart...be happy in the heart...be well in the heart...be at peace in your heart...be fully immersed in the blood of the Lord Jesus Christ...May the good Lord release you from the stronghold of all pressures of life in the heart...be blessed with the spirit of happiness in the heart...be set free from suffering in the heart...be healed from the spirit of illness of the heart...be healed in your body...be healed with good strength in your body...be happy in the body and heart...be healed in the name of the Lord Jesus Christ...Hallelujah; have light in your heart... be filled with that happy and comforting glory of the Lord Almighty in your heart...May the Holy Spirit take control of your heart and heal you...be comforted in the heart...rise above in the truth of the heart...be set free from evil of the heart...be healed in all goodness in the heart...In the powerful presence of the Holy Spirit, be cleansed in the heart...be happy in the heart and

body...be healed in the wonderful heart...be filled with the glory of God Almighty in your heart and life...be

healed in that powerful and saving name of the Lord Jesus
Christ. Amen.

Chapter 2

Heart protected

Psalm 18:2
"The LORD is my rock, my fortress and my deliverer; my God is my rock; in whom I take refuge. He is my shield and the horn of my salvation, my stronghold."

> * "I am strong in you my healer, O my Rock. You are my only everlasting strength. Re-establish me in your mercy and love. Favour me...cover me...immerse me in the blood of Jesus and cleanse my ailing body and spirit. Heal me Lord because I am weak and hopeless. Give me hope and strength...Come closer to my heart so that I may find rest in your mercy. Touch my heart with your sweetness and healing...Help me all the way...give me your joy and salvation because you are my only God and redeemer...you are my faithful and loving comforter."

Philippians 1:2
"Grace and peace to you from God our Father and the Lord Jesus Christ."

> * "I surrender to you my God...I surrender my broken body to you...I surrender my life and all that brings discomfort to my soul...I surrender my sadness, I surrender my aching heart, I surrender my cries and tears to you, I surrender all my worries, I surrender my illness to you, I surrender my hopelessness to you, I surrender my troubled family and children to you in this time of my trials and weakness, I surrender my life to

you in completeness, I surrender everything to you my saviour in the name of the Lord Jesus Christ my redeemer. You are the rock that is higher than I... I find rest and relief in you my hiding place...I surrender all to you my able God...Holy Jesus...merciful Spirit of God. I surrender!"

Psalm 25:16-18
"Turn to me and be gracious to me, for I am lonely and afflicted. The troubles of my heart have multiplied; free me from my anguish. Look upon my affliction and distress and take away all my sins."

  * Heavenly Father, make this burden in my life light for me. Free me from the stress that comes with illness. Liberate my soul from suffering. Help me Lord and remove disgrace. Walk with me and help me stand on solid ground. I feel humiliated, I feel so low, I feel unjustly treated by life. Everything is so wrong in my life. Help me Lord. I am so desperate. Take away this fearful and threatening humiliation of death and emptiness in the name of the Lord Jesus Christ. Comfort me with your healing power. Let there be life in my lungs...let there be adequate airflow in my lungs...Heal me Lord with your undefeated healing power. Make me strong. Help me to be steadfast in faith seeking your right hand.

Ephesians 6:10-11
"Finally be strong in the Lord and in his mighty power. Put on the full amour of God so that you can take your stand against the devil`s schemes."

  * I am alive...I am above and not beneath...I am living in the name of the Lord Jesus Christ. I will not die but I live to glorify his sovereignty, I live to uplift his

majestic name...I am free in the name of the Lord Jesus Christ...I am freed from the ugly spirit of disease and distortion of the body...I am freed from heartaches...I am freed from hopelessness...I am free in that glorious name of the Lord Jesus Christ...I live for the sake of my God...I am risen again through Jesus Christ. I am saved from the bizarre and weird spirit of death...God has favoured me...I am not without...God has forgiven me...God has given me life...God has loved me...God is good...God is powerful...God is full of love...God helps...God has given me his love in completeness...Yeah, God has protected me with the blood of the Lord Jesus Christ. God has healed me...God heals. God gives. God helps. God hears the prayers from my heart. God brings hope and relief to the soul...God makes my life easy and tolerable...My God is a God full of divine answers to my heart`s requests. God is awesome and ineffably sublime. God does not lie to my heart and life. God does not waver...he is true, faithful and steadfast... God is magnificent to me and my heart. God is beautiful, righteous and unconquerable. God heals...God is flawless. God is truthful in everything he says and does for my sake. My God delivers me. I am completely covered and protected with the blood of the Lord Jesus Christ. Devil get out of my life...get out of my heart...my heart belongs to Jesus Christ my Saviour...And in the Power in the blood of Jesus Christ, I command the devil to go...devil, you cannot touch me...you cannot hurt my body...you cannot come into my heart...my heart is the temple of the Holy Spirit...My heart belongs to Christ...My heart has the light and life of God...I am blessed in the heart and body...I overcome...I survive...I breakthrough...I am completely complete in the blood of the Lord Jesus Christ...My heart feels...my heart loves...my heart is glorious...I am made uniquely unique in the name and presence of my Lord Jesus Christ...I am healed in the blood of the Lamb...the blood of the Lord Jesus Christ that took away all my sins...My God has blessed me with a wonderful and perfect heart in that wonderful name of the Lord Jesus Christ. "God, you are marvellous and beautiful to me and I love you so much."

Ephesians 5:18

"Do not get drunk on wine, which leads to debauchery. Instead be filled with the Spirit. Speak to one another with psalms, hymns and spiritual songs. Sing and make music in your heart to the Lord, always giving thanks to God the Father for everything in the name of our Lord Jesus Christ."

* Dear Reader: Be healed in holiness in the name of the Lord Jesus Christ. Overcome the spirit of infirmity through the sacred power of God Almighty who gave you life on this land of the living. Surround yourself with love in this spiritual journey of healing. May the good Lord help you to remove fracas and factions in your life as you embark on this journey of healing with the Lord Jesus Christ...Surround yourself with God...Surround your heart with healing...Move along the moving and guidance of the Holy Spirit in your heart and body and it will all go well with you...Get rid of dilemmas; be surrounded by good things from God Almighty, Maker of heaven and earth. Do not be troubled in your heart...be at peace...be a good person in truth and in spirit because your life is not dilapidated...Love the Lord your God wholeheartedly because he has given you back your life...

* Tell the Lord this; "Lord I heartily love you for being my God, my only God."

* Yes, my friend, you will be fine...You will live your life in good health...Your heart is made perfectly strong...Be healed in the glorious name of the Lord Jesus Christ. Be healed and be holy because your God is a holy God.

Zephaniah 3:14
"Sing, O Daughter of Zion; shout aloud, O Israel! Be glad and rejoice with all your heart, O daughter of Jerusalem."

* I have hope. I am not afraid, the Lord is with me, the Lord God, Maker of heaven and earth will heal me forever and ever in the name of the Lord Jesus Christ. My throat is being healed in the powerful name of the Lord Jesus Christ. I have no more painful lumps...My heart is being healed. My whole body is being touched and healing completely in his great name. I am regaining strength in that powerful name of the Lord Jesus Christ. I am thankful with all my heart and soul.

Matthew 5:10
"Happy are those who are persecuted because they do what God requires; the Kingdom of heaven belongs to them."

* Heart; overcome victimization in the name of the Lord Jesus Christ...Be triumphant dear heart in this powerful name...be freed from affliction of High Blood Pressure...Be well in the veins and blood...Heart; receive justice over all wrongs and be happy...receive contentment...may the Lord God Almighty rise above for you in the name of the Lord Jesus Christ. Heart; the Lord your God who loves you will shame all those who mistreat you...you will rise above dear heart in the

saving name of the Lord Jesus Christ...Heart; do not be offended, the Lord Jesus Christ died for your salvation and by his blood you are healed...do not feel ill-treated dear heart, be a winner in the blood of the Lord Jesus Christ...be healed and conquer in the name of the Lord Jesus Christ...Be at peace in his saving name...may his protecting presence fill you dear heart...Be successful in the power of the Holy Spirit...Be healed in his sovereign power...feel majestic dear heart...Be confident...You are a winner because God is within you and for you and will always comfort your spirit. You live in perfect happiness in the giving name of the Lord Jesus Christ. You are surrounded by his saving glory dear heart. Darkness cannot win over you dear heart...Be healed in the powerful name of the Lord Jesus Christ....Hallelujah; you are healed in your blood...you are healed in your heart...you are healed in your veins...you are healed in your arteries...you healed with a wonderful healing of God Almighty in the name of Jesus Christ...You are cleansed in your heart, blood and brain...you are cleansed in your body...you are protected from demise...you are protected in your heart, body, soul, mind, blood, veins and arteries...You are protected from the top of your head and all the way to the soles of your feet...You are healed from High Blood Pressure...you are healed in that wonderful name of the Lord Jesus Christ...You are healed from low blood pressure...you are healed from all diseases of the blood, veins and arteries...you are healed in that wonderful name of the Lord Jesus Christ...Live your life in peace all the days of your life in the name of the Lord Jesus Christ.

Hallelujah.

Thank you Jesus Christ, My Saviour and my Best
Friend.... Thank you Father God...thank you for the cross
that has made a difference in the lives of mankind and all
creation. Thank you Holy Spirit, you are God and you are
good.

Amen.

End.

Bibliography

Powered by the Finger of God, Holy Spirit, living and active.

Holy Bible NIV

Good News Bible (American Bible Society)